Battling Head & Neck Cancer With Nutrition

Heather Gabbert, MS, RD, LD, CD
Kathy Beach, RN
Christopher M. Lee, MD

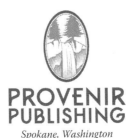

PROVENIR
PUBLISHING
Spokane, Washington

www.provenirpublishing.com

Battling Head And Neck Cancer With Nutrition

The authors, editors, and publisher have made every effort to provide accurate information. However, they are not responsible for errors, omissions, or for any outcomes related to the use of contents of this book and take no responsibility for the use of the products and procedures described. The editors, editorial board, sponsoring organization, and publisher do not assume responsibility for the statements expressed by the authors in their contributions. Treatments and side effects described in this book may not be applicable to all people; likewise, some people may require a different treatment than described herein due to individual circumstances. Drugs and medical devices are discussed, but may have limited availability controlled by the Food and Drug Administration (FDA) for use only in a research study or clinical trial. Research, clinical practice, and government relations often change the accepted standard in the field. When consideration is being given to use of any drug in a clinical setting, the health care provider or reader is responsible for determining the optimal treatment for an individual patient and is responsible for reviewing the most up-to-date recommendations on dose, precautions, and contra indications, and determining the appropriate usage for the product. This is especially important in the case of drugs that are new or seldom used.

Published by Provenir Publishing, LLC, P. O. Box 211, Greenacres, WA 99016-0211

Production Credits

Lead Editor: Christopher Lee

Production Director: Amy Harman

Art Director and Illustration: Micah Harman

Cover Design: Micah Harman

Printing History: April 2013, First Edition.

This book is dedicated to our patients and their families,
who inspire us every day in their cancer fight.

Contents

Head and neck cancer (cancer of the mouth, tongue, and/or throat) is a malignant neoplasm originating from abnormal cells arising in tissues forming the pancreas. The most common type of head and neck cancer is squamous cell carcinoma, which accounts for 95% of these tumors.

Head and neck cancer is known to be an aggressive type of malignancy, and requires in many cases surgery, radiation, and chemotherapy treatments. Because of the aggressive nature of this diagnosis, treatment of this cancer requires a multidisciplinary team of physicians and care providers, including specialists in dietary needs and nutrition.

It is very common for patients with a cancer diagnosis to have many questions about nutrition and diet. In fact, this is one of the main ways that you (or your loved one) can aid yourself in the battle with cancer. The cancer can inhibit your body's ability to heal, decrease your energy, and decrease your immune system. By optimizing diet and nutrition, research has shown that outcomes of surgery, radiation, and chemotherapy are improved. This leads to improved cure rates, better cancer treatment outcomes, and greater ability for the body to heal and rebound from the effects of cancer therapy.

CHAPTER ONE

Focusing On Nutrition

You have been diagnosed with cancer in the head and neck area. You may feel out of control and unsettled right now, but I'm here to tell you how you can be a little bit in control of what may feel like an out of control situation. What you choose to eat can have a strong impact on fighting this cancer. Your immune

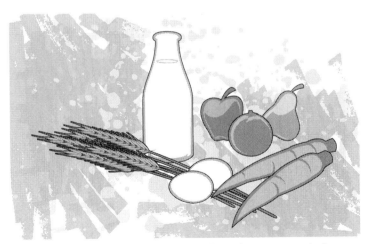

Focusing on nutrition can be the best thing that you can do for yourself during cancer therapy.

1

system is what fights off illnesses and disease. By making the best choices nutritionally, you can maximize your immune system's fighting potential, making you the best cancer fighter you can be. It's all about boosting your immune system, fighting inflammation and decreasing challenges to your immune system so it can focus on the current battle at hand. The information you walk away with today isn't just for here and now, it's for life and long-term health.

CHAPTER TWO

Immune Boosting Nutrition

Make every bite count. Well, almost every bite. I like to follow the 80/20 rule. Eighty percent of the time you should make every bite count. Make the best choice for what you decide to fuel your body with. So often we are on the go, or in a hurry, and making unconscious decisions regarding our nutritional intake. Think about it. Is what you are eating doing anything for your body and your fight against cancer? If not, maybe you should think about making some changes in your food selections. That's not to say you can't enjoy those foods that, let's be honest, aren't good for you but they sure taste good and make you feel happy. You can. These are the foods that you have only around 20% of the time. Enjoying birthday celebrations, dessert out with girlfriends, poker night with the guys, whatever it may be, will most likely involve chips, dips and drink choices that you seldom consume. It's OK to enjoy these moments. Make a conscious effort to eat the best you can most of the time, so you can enjoy these special moments and the "not so good" nutrition choices that accompany these occasions without the guilt. It's all part of a healthy eating experience. It's all part of life, as is this current fight you've got on your hands.

Mainly, regarding your diet, the focus should lie on getting back to the basics. Grandma was right! You are what you eat! Having whole foods and less processed foods is where it's at. When buying boxed/convenience foods, select those with less ingredients. Take ice cream for example. It can be a source of protein and calcium, but also has a high content of fat; therefore, only have it occasionally. What I want you to look at, though, is how many ingredients went into the making of it. Buy the ice cream containing only five ingredients or so. Breyers All Natural is a good example of this. I'm not saying eat ice cream all the time, but it is okay sometimes, especially if there are no chemicals/preservatives added to it. This was just an example. In general, focus on eating whole grains, dark and brightly colored fruits and vegetables, plant proteins, lean animal protein sources, fish (especially those high in Omega-3 fatty acids), and other good fats which are listed below. The idea is to balance out carbs and protein at each meal, mini meal or snack. Also by incorporating the good fats into your diet, this will also help in sparing the protein you take in for healing and repair.

Whole Grains

When choosing whole grain foods, select those that

have been the least processed or broken down. Some examples of whole grains include: brown rice, wild rice, whole wheat pasta, quinoa, quinoa pasta, high fiber cereals (hot or cold) containing 5 grams or more fiber per serving, and breads made from whole grain flour, having 3 grams of fiber or more per slice. Whole grain flour being the first ingredient listed. Whole grains have complex carbohydrates in them which are needed by our bodies for energy. They also have protein in them. Quinoa, for example, has 5-8 grams of protein per ½ cup. Give it a try if you haven't already.

Produce

It is recommended that 5 or more servings of fruit and vegetables be consumed each day. This is challenging for a lot of people. What I recommend is to add a fruit or vegetable to every meal, mini meal or snack eaten during the day. Try to eat small meals, every 3 hours or so. At each of these add a serving of produce. Aim for 5 servings a day of dark or brightly colored produce.

Some of the best choices include:

- *Broccoli, cauliflower, brussels sprouts, kale and bok choy.* These are called cruciferous vegetables and they contain isothiocyanates, specifically Indole-3-Carbinol. This is a cancer fighting compound and should be consumed on a daily basis!

- Berries of all varieties

- Carrots and orange colored produce for the

carotenoids.

- Red grapes for the resveratrol

- Green leafies

- Tomatoes

This is a short list of some of the most powerful cancer fighting produce available at grocery stores. It is highly recommended you have your own garden if you can, and grow produce organically. Another thing that should always be mentioned when discussing produce is to wash it in a vinegar and water solution. Wash produce using a solution of 1 Tablespoon vinegar (any kind) in 4 cups of water. This will help to pull off 95-99% of the cancer-causing pesticides used in the farming of the produce. For the thin skinned fruits and hard to wash vegetables, it is better to go organic because it is difficult to completely clean these off. This decreases challenges to your immune system, eliminating one less thing to worry about.

Plant Proteins

Foods of plant origin are high in fiber, vitamins, minerals, antioxidants, beneficial plant compounds, and prebiotic fibers to help support healthy intestinal bacteria balance. Plant based foods are the basis for an anti-inflammatory diet. Beans, legumes, lentils, nuts, seeds, soy foods—these are all sources of protein coming from a plant source. GO FOR IT! Add these to your salads, soups, chili's, or make a bean burger, etc. The list goes on and on.

Animal Proteins

Protein from animal sources is allowed also, but be sure to buy leaner cuts of meat, chicken and other poultry with no skin, and go organic when it comes to purchasing red meat and dairy products containing fat. Buy grass fed cattle because it is higher in Omega-3 fatty acids which are anti-inflammatory. Animal foods, in general, contain higher amounts of Omega-6 fatty acids which are pro-inflammatory so the goal is to decrease intake of animal based foods, while we increase intake of plant based foods and fish, especially those high in Omega-3 fats. (sources listed below) *NOTE: Avoid processed/cured meats due to their nitrite/ nitrate content. This is a cancer causing agent used in hams, deli meats, hot dogs, bacon and sausages. Use a nitrate-free product such as Hormel Natural Selections. It can be found in the deli meat section of the grocery store.*

List Of Protein Foods

Beans, legumes, lentils – typical serving size is 1/4 cup which equals 7 grams protein. Increase bean intake – try hummus spread, made from garbanzo beans (aka chickpeas).
Nuts, seeds – 1/4 cup = 7 grams protein. If nuts and seeds are not tolerated, grind nuts into a spread at your local grocery store. The nut grinders are usually found in the "Health Food" section of the grocery stores by the "All Natural" items.

Milks and spreads/nut butter made from plant foods – almond milk, soy milk, soy yogurt, grind any nut to make a nut butter at your local grocery store.

Fish – especially wild caught salmon, tuna, halibut, mackerel and rainbow trout, for their Omega-3 fatty acid content. Omega-3s, as stated previously, are a natural anti-inflammatory and should be consumed 2-3 times per week. Other fish do not contain high levels of Omega-3s, however, are lean protein sources, with 4 ounces being a serving of fish it provides 28 grams of protein.

Eggs are a high quality protein – each egg has about 5-7 grams of protein. Suggest having 5 eggs a week and unlimited egg whites.

Chicken and turkey – no skin, are lean protein sources. Each ounce has 7 grams protein.

LEAN cuts of red meat –sirloin, ground sirloin for burgers versus ground chuck, and flank steak for fajitas, for example, would be okay for consumption. Also, look for grass-fed cattle as this meat will have more Omega-3s versus the inflammatory Omega-6s. The American Institute of Cancer Research (AICR) recommends limiting intake of red meat, to about 3 servings per week.

Greek yogurt – has about 12-14 grams protein in it and the live cultures (probiotics) will help to normalize gut flora and promote bacteria balance in the intestines.

Low or no-fat dairy – skim milk, 1% milk, low-fat, skim mozzarella, etc. When buying a fat-containing animal product it is recommended to go organic. Look for this statement or something similar on the label, "No hormones or antibiotics were given to this animal or used in the making of this product." Keep in mind when buying fat-containing animal foods: hormones, and toxins given to the animal are stored in the fat of the animal. The fattier the animal food, the more likely you are to consume the bad things stored in the fat of the animal. Safer to go organic when it comes to fat-containing animal products. Wise to spend your money on organic meats and dairy products.

Good Fats

Lowering dietary intake of Omega-6 fats (mostly animal foods) while raising intake of Omega-3 fats will help to shift the body into "anti-inflammatory" mode. What are good sources of Omega-3s? High Omega-3 foods include wild caught salmon, tuna, halibut, mackerel and rainbow trout. Also, foods of plant origin will have less Omega-6 fats and some Omega-3s like walnuts and flaxseed oil. Extra virgin olive oil, canola oil and coconut oil are examples of good fats as are avocados, nuts and seeds. Daily intake of a ¼–½ of an avocado is recommended.

CHAPTER THREE

Balance, Timing, And Planning

Fueling your body consistently all day long, every day, will help you maintain an even keel throughout the day and avoid blood sugar peaks and valleys. By staying on an even keel all day you will provide needed support to your immune system so that it can work at its best potential. Blood sugar stabilization is key. The number one thing I hear from patients is, "I don't eat breakfast." Or, "My whole life I've never eaten breakfast." Now is the time for that to change. Try to consume calories, whether it's eating or drinking, within an hour of waking. You need to wake the body up and let it know that nutrition is on the way. If you're not doing this, it is very likely that your metabolism will slow down.

Another very important thing to remember is that caffeine is an appetite suppressant. I have countless people tell me, "I just drink black coffee all morning and I'm not hungry for anything until about 4:00 in the afternoon." The reason one can go so long without having an appetite is due in part to the caffeine intake as it is suppressing the hunger cue. In actuality, you are slowing down the metabolism. What you need now is a well-oiled machine and to stay revved up to support weight maintenance as well as your immune system. We are addressing weight management and immune-boosting nutrition. To continue boosting the immune system and support your cancer fighting body, I suggest trying to eat every 3 hours, trying never to go longer than 4 hours between intake. This will help to support blood sugar stability all day long and keep you and your immune system energized.

Imagine this: your body is a wood stove. You want to keep the fire burning all day long so you need logs (protein foods) and kindling (carbohydrates) every few hours. Why do this? The answer is simple. If your body doesn't have a consistent source of fuel, it will think "uh-oh, I don't have anything coming in", and begin to work its magic in fueling your body, slowing things down if you will and eventually pulling from energy stores. You have stored energy in your muscles and when not properly nourished you may begin to breakdown muscle. A good way to gauge muscle loss is to look at your arms. Look for atrophy (shrinking muscle mass). Notice if there is any muscle or fat loss. Of course, monitor your weight.

It is okay to lose a little bit of weight but you want to avoid significant weight loss during your cancer treatment. Your radiation team will be following your weight status weekly. The registered dietitian on the team will be alerted if you should experience significant weight loss, change in nutritional status, and/or begin to be more symptomatic. A nutrition consult would be beneficial to address symptoms and give you ways to manage them.

CHAPTER FOUR

Treating The Symptoms Of Cancer Or Treatment

Symptoms often associated with radiation to the head and neck region include: dry mouth, mouth tenderness, sore throat, painful swallowing, difficulty swallowing, and intolerance to foods that are either too hot or too cold. During radiation, the body will naturally send lubrication in the form of a sticky thick mucus-like saliva, as well as send inflammation to the radiation site. Sure the body is trying to heal this area, but it can make it very difficult to swallow when this site is in the head and neck region. To manage the sticky, thick mucus-like saliva, it is best to stay hydrated. Drink water or tea constantly to provide yourself with adequate fluids. This will help to thin out the secretions and make it easier to expectorate

NURSE'S NOTE:

If nausea is an issue, it may help to keep a food diary. This will help you decide which foods to eliminate during therapy to help alleviate side effects.

(cough up).

Dry Mouth/Tender Mouth

• Sip water and teas frequently throughout the day to moisten mouth.

• Limit caffeine and alcohol intake as they tend to be a diuretic and pull fluid out of the body.

• Use a non alcohol containing mouthwash such as Biotene.

• Have water/water bottle with you at all times—take frequent sips.

• Consume moist foods such as stews, casseroles, soups, and fruits.

• Suck on ice chips, popsicles, or make slushies if cold temperature foods are desired and tolerated.

• Use broth, gravies, sauces, yogurt, silken tofu (moist and creamy), warm water, juices, milk or dairy alternatives, and coconut milk to moisten foods.

• Eat soft foods such as yogurt, all natural ice cream, oatmeal, pudding, Cream Of Wheat, Malt-O-Meal, even cooked vegetables such as cauliflower can be mashed to make "mock mashed potatoes."

• Use olive oil, canola oil, and/or coconut oil to make foods slippery and easier to swallow.

• Avoid crunchy textured foods, tough meats, and raw

vegetables.

NURSE'S NOTE:

If you use gum, mints, or hard candy to help with dry mouth, choose sugar free as sugar aids in the growth of yeast.

• Chew xylitol based gum. Xylitol is a sugar-free sweetener and does not promote tooth decay. This is available in most grocery stores down the "health food" or "all natural" sections of the store.

• Use a humidifier in your room at night to keep the air moist.

• Moisten lips frequently with lip balm, Aquafor, cocoa butter or olive oil.

Painful/Difficulty Swallowing

During radiation treatment, it can become increasingly difficult to eat. The first few weeks you may think, "Oh, OK, I can do this, a little Magic Mouthwash and I can eat." Then it may be something like, "Ouch, it's really hurting to swallow solid foods, I'll stick to liquids or soft foods like yogurt, pudding, ice cream..." This throat pain is only going to get worse.

While we want you to continue attempts at swallowing, this can be done with sips of water and caloric liquids such as juices, popsicles, smoothies, protein shakes or slushies, etc. One simple thing you can do is drink a high calorie nutritional supplement. There are many to choose from and you can even make your own using whey or plant based protein powder. One calorie dense drink I do recommend to gain weight after a big weight loss or to prevent this from happening is Carnation VHC (Very High Calorie). This drink, unlike Ensure or Boost, is not available retail. You can ask at your cancer care facility or you can possibly contact a local home health company on your own and ask them if they carry this formula or something similar.

I suggest you drink this throughout the day at a ¼ cup dose (equivalent to ¼ can), 4 times per day, refrigerating the formula in between drinks. This will equal one can total per day which is 560 calories. This can help to maintain weight, or at the very least minimize weight loss. *What we don't want to happen is significant weight loss during cancer therapy.* Weight loss greatly weakens your nutritional status and your fighting power.

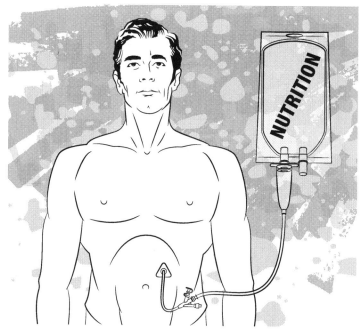

A feeding tube can become a "life-line" for you during radiation treatment if excessive weight loss is a problem.

To prevent weight loss and an impaired nutritional status, the use of a feeding tube is highly recommended for some patients. A feeding tube is a necessary, mostly temporary, means of nourishing your body. It's plain and simple, if you can't swallow your food/liquids you can't meet your nutritional needs. Be proactive and have a feeding tube placed if needed (of course this should be discussed with your health providers to determine if this is best for you).

Once treatment is underway and your esophagus becomes inflamed from therapy, it can potentially be very painful to have the tube placed using an endoscope down your throat. For some patients, it is protocol that a feeding tube be placed prior to the start of radiation treatment. Tubes are placed using a variety of procedures. Some physicians only have the PEG (percutaneous endoscopic gastrostomy) placed while others have tubes placed directly into the stomach using radiologic guidance. This is also an option once treatment has started, but the earlier it is placed, the quicker you can start to get additional needed calories into your body.

Be sure to discuss feeding tube options with your radiation team, specifically, your doctor, registered dietician and nurse. There are different ways to administer feedings through the feeding tube. They are called: bolus, gravity and pump feeds. The only thing that can go in the feeding tube is liquid. There are pre-made formulas like Boost, Ensure, Fibersource, Carnation VHC, or you can make your own mixture if you like.

High Impact Snacks

Consuming foods that provide a power packed

punch to oxidants and have a high impact upon every bite is where it's at! Eating snacks that are high in calories and protein, preferably from a plant source and a source of good fats is the best way to go.

Some Examples Include:

Trail mix – 1/4 –1/2 cup mixture of nuts and dried fruit will give you good fats, carbs, fiber and protein.

Hummus (garbanzo bean spread) – 2 TBSP on whole wheat pita or with 6–10 baby carrots.

A *nut butter spread* – peanut butter, almond butter, etc. – 2 TBSP on whole grain bread/bagel thin/brown rice crackers, etc.

Protein powder infused smoothie – use whey protein or rice protein. Add to fruit smoothie. Example of ingredients could be: berries, greek yogurt or almond milk, and protein powder. You can add more fruits and veggies to really pack a punch! Do not juice as we want the pulp from the produce because it is loaded with cancer fighting nutrients.

Greek yogurt – has higher concentration of protein. Add a whole grain and or fruit which will work as pre-biotics. Pre-biotics are food for the probiotics that are in the yogurt. The probiotics help to normalize gut flora, therefore, better supporting the immune system.

Chapter Five

Supplements

The AICR (American Institute of Cancer Research) has made a recommendation to take minimal supplements while increasing nutrient density of your food intake. We do know from recent research that many of us are deficient in vitamin D. Vitamin D deficiencies are linked with cancer, MS, depression, insomnia, aches/pains, etc. Getting your vitamin D tested is highly recommended and from there it can be determined if vitamin D3 supplementation is necessary.

Fish oil is often recommended because of its anti-inflammatory properties. 1500-3000 mg/day Omega-3s is recommended each day. The Omega-3s are DHA and EPA. Look for the content of these on the back of the supplement bottle. Concentrations vary greatly so be sure to take adequate amounts. If scheduled to have surgery, be sure to tell your surgeon and all physicians involved you are taking fish oil. It is recommended that fish oil be stopped prior to procedures as it thins out the blood.

A multivitamin a day is usually appropriate. Go

Nurse's Note:
Ask your doctor or nurse about nutrition supplements.

over contents of it with your registered dietitian and/ or doctor.

A fiber supplement such as acacia fiber, is beneficial if you are prone to constipation or extreme cycles of diarrhea then constipation. If you have increased fiber in your diet by incorporating whole grains, fruits and vegetables, supplementation may not be necessary.

The great debate continues on whether to take antioxidant supplementation during treatment or not. Recommendations vary greatly on what is allowed or not allowed during treatment and you will need to discuss this with your oncologists. One thing I tell patients is to listen to your body. You have a mind/body connection and need to listen to it. If you feel confident that something is working for you, then do it. Don't do some supplement just because someone told you about it and it worked for them or because that is what you read on the internet. Of course you will get tons of advice at every turn, but take time to digest it all and figure out what works for you. Rather than focusing on supplementation for added nutrients, it is better to focus on maximizing your nutrient intake through food. You can go to *www.ORACvalues.com*. ORAC stands for oxygen radical absorbance capacity, which is the antioxidant power of foods. *ORACvalues.com* is a comprehensive database of foods and their antioxidant levels. Some things high in ORAC are: parsley, blueberries and cinnamon. Check out the website to see what others are high in ORAC values!

NOTE: *Always discuss all meds, natural supplements, vitamins and minerals with your doctor to assure nothing is compromising your treatment.*

Recommended Resources

Recommended Books

Eating Well Through Cancer – distributed by Merck

The Cancer Lifeline Cookbook – by Kimberly Mathai MS, RD, with Ginny Smith

The Cancer–Fighting Kitchen and One Bite at a Time – by Rebecca Katz

In the above-mentioned books you will find whole-foods based recipes and wonderfully helpful nutrition information.

Online Resources

I would like to address the world of online information. You will see many things on the computer. "Googling" has become a way of life but be careful in what sites you go to. There is one theory found online that gets brought up the most. It is the theory that "sugar feeds cancer." I want you to remember one thing: anything growing inside of us will be fueled by what we are fueled by. Our main energy source is glucose. This is sugar. As stated before, follow the 80/20 rule of thumb with regards to diet and nutrition. Most definitely do not avoid fruits and whole grains in hopes of depriving your body of sugar or in hopes of starving the tumor. Keep the focus on balance of carbohydrates, proteins, and good fats. Eat whole grains, bright or dark colored produce, plant proteins, lean or lower fat animal proteins, and good fats.

Recommended Websites

There are numerous websites to view. So much so it can be overwhelming. Below is a list of credible websites.

www.caring4cancer.com/go/cancer/nutrition – the side effects management section is written by a registered dietitian.

www.cancer.org

www.cancerrd.com

http://oralcancerfoundation.org

www.cancer.gov/cancertopics/wyntk/oral

www.nlm.nih.gov/medlineplus/oralcancer.html

www.aicr.org/site/PageServer

www.mypyramidtracker.gov/planner/

www.oralcancerfoundation.org/dental/xerostomia. htm – information on dry mouth.

www.foodnews.org – for the Dirty Dozen annual report on produce.

www.consumerlabs.com – to review your supplement. See if it passed quality testing.

www.ORACvalues.com – to review antioxidant levels of foods.

www.livestrong.org

www.asha.org/public/speech/disorders/Swallowing-Probs.htm – American Speech Language and Hearing Institute.

Journal

_____
_____
_____
_____
_____
_____
_____
_____
_____
_____
_____
_____
_____
_____
_____
_____
_____
_____
_____
_____
_____
_____
_____
_____
_____

JOURNAL

Common Cancer Terms

Adjuvant therapy: Treatment used after the main treatment (i.e., after radiation or surgery). As an example, chemotherapy or radiation may be given after surgery to increase the chance of cure.

Base of Tongue: The part of the tongue you can't see that extends down the back of the throat.

Benign tumor: An abnormal growth of cells that is NOT cancer and forms an abnormal lump.

Biopsy: A procedure in which a small piece of tissue is taken for examination by a pathologist to see if cancer is present or not.

Buccal mucosa: The soft lining on the inside of the cheeks.

Cancer: A term used when cells with damaged or abnormal DNA start to grow out of control.

Chemotherapy: Medicine usually given by an IV to stop cancer cells from dividing and spreading.

Computerized Axial Tomography: Otherwise known as a CT scan. This is a picture taken to evaluate the anatomy of the head and neck in three dimensions.

Deoxyribonucleic Acid: Otherwise known as DNA. This is something found in every cell of the body. It is what programs a cell to do specific functions.

Ethmoid sinus: An air space found between the eyebrows and below the bone.

Feeding tube: A flexible tube placed in the stomach through which nutrition can be given.

Gastro esophageal Reflux Disease (GERD): A condition in which stomach acid moves up into the esophagus and causes a burning sensation.

Grade: Term that helps describe the aggressiveness of tumor cells.

Hard palate: Roof of the mouth.

Histology: A description of the cancer cells which can distinguish what part of the body the cells originated from.

Hypopharynx: The lowest part of the throat above the larynx that helps to keep food and fluids from entering the lungs.

Intensity Modulated Radiation Therapy: Also known as IMRT. A complex type of radiation therapy where many beams are used. It spares surrounding normal tissues and treats the cancer with more precision.

Laryngectomy: The term used for surgically removing the voice box or larynx.

Larynx: The voice box (contains your vocal cords).

Localized cancer: Cancer that has not spread to another part of the body.

Leukoplakia: A whitish patch inside the mouth.

Lymph nodes: Bean shaped structures that are the "filter" of the body. The fluid that passes through them is called lymph fluid and filters unwanted materials like cancer cells, bacteria, and viruses.

Malignant: A tumor that is cancer.

Maxillary sinuses: Air spaces behind the cheeks and above the jaw.

Metastasis: The spread of cancer cells to other parts of the body such as the lungs or bones.

Nasopharynx: The air pocket between the eyes and behind the nose.

Neck dissection: Surgery of the neck that removes lymph nodes to check for spread of cancer.

Neoadjuvant therapy: Chemotherapy or radiation that is given before surgery (or radiation) to help shrink the tumor.

Oropharynx: Area made up of the soft palate, uvula, tonsils, base of the tongue, and the walls of the pharynx.

Osteoradionecrosis: Damage to the bone caused by radiation effecting blood flow to the bone.

Otolaryngologist: A doctor that specializes in ear, nose, and throat (ENT).

Palliative treatment: Treatment that helps relieve the symptoms of cancer, such as pain, but does not cure the disease.

Pathologist: A doctor trained to recognize tumor cells as benign or cancerous.

Pharynx: Area of the throat.

Positron Emission Tomography: Also known as a PET scan. This test is used to look at cell metabolism to recognize areas in the body where the cancer may be hiding.

Pyriform sinuses: The air space on either side of the larynx (or voice box).

Radiation therapy: Invisible high energy beams that can shrink or kill cancer cells.

Recurrence: When cancer comes back after treatment.

Remission: Partial or complete disappearance of the signs and symptoms of cancer. This is not necessarily a cure.

Risk factors: Environmental and genetic factors that increase our chance of getting cancer.

Side effects: Unwanted effects of treatment such as hair loss, burns or rash on the skin, sore throat, etc.

Simulation: Mapping session where radiation is planned. If the doctor will be using a mask for your treatment, this is the time it will be custom fit for your face.

Soft palate: Back area that connects to the roof of the mouth and makes up the soft part (this is where the uvula hangs from).

Sphenoid sinuses: Air spaces behind the sphenoid bone.

Staging: Tests that help to determine if the cancer has spread to lymph nodes or other organs.

Tonsils: Soft tissue on both sides of the throat. Tonsils are part of the lymphatic system.

Tumor: A new growth of tissue which forms a lump on or inside the body that may or may not be cancerous.

Uvula: The soft piece of tissue that hangs down in the back of the throat.

About The Authors

Heather Gabbert, MS, RD, LD, CD: Heather attended Southern Illinois University at Carbondale and graduated with her Master's Degree in Dietetics in 1995. She has been a Registered Dietitian (RD) for 17 years and has lived in different areas of the country throughout the years, in each place, gaining valuable experience in the field of dietetics. She has worked with cancer patients since 1998 when she began working at Cancer Treatment Centers of America. She continued to work intermittently for CTCA throughout the many years she has been a practitioner. Heather moved to Spokane, Washington, from Chicago, Illinois, in 2007 where she works as an RD for Cancer Care Northwest and a home health company. Professionally, Heather's passion lies in working with cancer patients and promoting wellness and disease prevention for all.

Heather is a member of Academy of Nutrition and Dietetics (AND), Washington State Academy of Nutrition and Dietetics (WSAND), and Greater Spokane Dietetics Association (GSDA). She served for two years as Media Representative and board member for WSAND and GSDA. Heather has authored a book, been a contributing writer, written articles and was a blogger for StepUpSpokane, highlighting nutrition and wellness. She is a member of AND's DPG groups: Oncology, Business Communications and Entrepreneurs, Dietitians in Integrative Medicine, and Sports, Cardio and Wellness Nutrition (SCAN) group.

Heather most enjoys time spent with her two children. She also enjoys life as a Zumba instructor, exerciser and most memorable activities are her first half marathon and participating in an adventure race, which involved trail-running, biking and kayaking.

Kathy Beach, RN: Kathy graduated with her RN degree in 1993. She decided to get a degree in nursing after her mother was diagnosed with breast cancer.

She spent sixteen years in hospital nursing where she worked on a wide range of units from Medical Oncology to Outpatient Surgery. For the past 4 years, she has focused her energy in oncology and radiation oncology with Cancer Care Northwest in Spokane, WA. She loves her work and finds the patients she cares for and their families to be extremely inspiring.

Christopher M. Lee, MD: Dr. Lee is a practicing Radiation Oncologist and is the Director of Research for Cancer Care Northwest and The Gamma Knife of Spokane (Spokane, WA). Dr. Lee graduated cum laude in Biochemistry from Brigham Young University in 1997 which included a summer research fellowship at Harvard University and Brigham and Women's Hospital. He subsequently attended Saint Louis University School of Medicine where he received his M.D. with Distinction in Research degree. He completed four additional years of specialty training in Radiation Oncology at the Huntsman Cancer Hospital and University of Utah Medical Center during which he was given multiple national awards. Dr. Lee has actively pursued both basic science and clinical research throughout his career. He continues to be a proliferative author of scientific papers and regularly gives presentations on radiotherapy technique and the use of targeted radiation in the care of patients with head and neck (throat), brain, breast, gynecologic, and prostate malignancies.

Made in the USA
Charleston, SC
05 August 2013